Water Diet:

Body Cleansing And Weight Loss With The Help Of Water

Table of Contents

Introduction

You must drink water daily. It is good for both your skin and body. Even, if you find it difficult to consume half glass of water half hour before your meal every time, you can replace the calorie-loaded drinks such as juice or soda with a plain glass of water.

Cellulite is not everyone's favorite topic. Loving your body is a big art. It does not matter if you have a few pockets and some dimples to spare on your thighs. Water can help you reduce it.

The human body must always be kept hydrated. The muscles start losing their elasticity with the diminishing water content. With this worse development, the muscles get tight and might get spasms as well.

Many people believe in applying various fruits and vegetables on their skins to nourish it which is a good practice and makes the skin healthier and more glowing. Along with it, what you eat also contributes towards the nourishment of your skin. That's why a healthy diet with lots of water and lot of fresh veggies and fruits must be consumed.

Chapter 1 – Water Diet to Get Wrinkle Free Skins

Every organ, tissue, and cell of the human body requires water to survive and to carry out the tasks correctly. For example, your body uses water to remove wastes, maintain its temperature, and lubricate the joints and hydrate the muscles. Your skin requires water as well.

Drinking lots of organic, clean water is an inevitable part of maintaining both of your health and skin. As the human body gets older, it loses its ability to retain water and moisture in it. It results in dehydration of the body. These effects can be seen in the form of wrinkles on the skin.

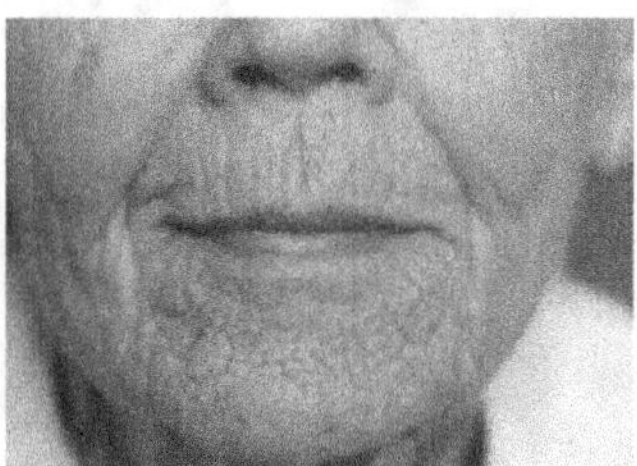

Dehydrated skin also does not have the ability to repair itself. Also, it is unable to generate new cells. It results in the appearance of the signs of aging in human bodies. Thus, hydrating your body can reduce these effects. You must hydrate your skin from inside and outside.

In this chapter, we are discussing the methods of hydrating your skin and reducing the appearance of wrinkles on it with water: Let's read together!

Aging Skin:

Human skin undergoes various changes as it ages. The complexion of the skin loses its firmness and bounce due to the decrease in production of collagen in your skin with age. It results in a loss of hyaluronic acid and elastin. Both of these elements are essential to retain moisture in your skin and to ward off any damage.

Also, your lifestyle and the environmental factors such as smoking and exposure to direct sunlight also affect your skin adversely when it is aged.

Effects of Moisture Loss:

The skin becomes flaky and cracked as it loses its moisture. You may need topical products to provide necessary moisture to your skin, so it stays alive. Dry skin saps the moisture of the cells and looks unhealthy. It results in shriveling up of the cells and thus, the wrinkles become more prominent.

Water retains moisture in your skin and helps it performing its functions properly. Also, the adequate intake of water keeps the cells working accurately. It also makes your skin appear smooth and supple.

Adequate Water Intake:

Experts recommend an average human being to consume more or less eight glasses of pure organic and clean water every day, as per the report of the National Institute of Health. However, your body may demand more water if you sweat a lot, or you are exercising.

Also, if you live in a humid, dry environment, the water requirement of your body will be higher than other people. Certain kinds of meditation may also dehydrate your body and skin. Therefore, it is pertinent to talk to your physician if you are not sure about the exact amount of water you need to take every day as per the requirements of your body.

Considerations:

Water is an excellent supplement to maintain and retain the level of moisture in your skin. But it is only the primary thing. You need to go some extra miles to deal with the wrinkles in your skin.

You must take a balanced diet to maintain the glow and freshness of your skin. It includes the proper amount of fresh fruits and vegetables, a certain amount of proteins and lots of water.

You must drink water daily. It is good for both your skin and body. It fills your stomach and makes you eat less especially if you are regular in taking it before your meal every day. Thus, you start losing weight without holding up to any particular diet plan. Here are some of the outstanding greens that are essential for your skin:

Cucumbers: The water content of cucumber is 96.7%. It is the only solid food that contains this much water in it. You can serve it with hummus, eat in slices, or make part of a salad. You can even pump up its moisture content by blending it up with ice cubes, mint, and nonfat yogurt. It will make up soup for you.

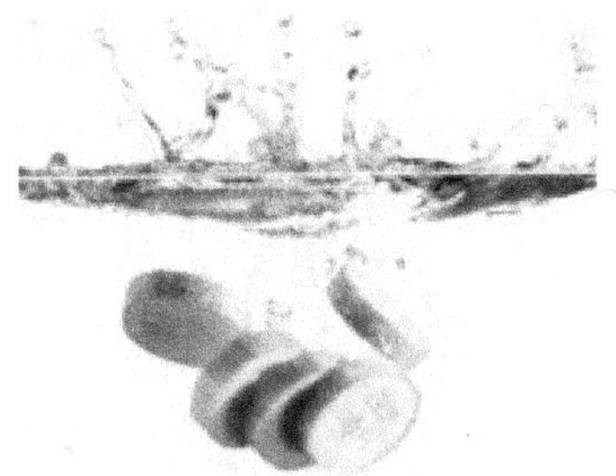

Green peppers: all bell peppers have high water texture, yet green bell peppers are on the top with 93.9% water content. They make a great addition to your salad with the sharp, hot taste.

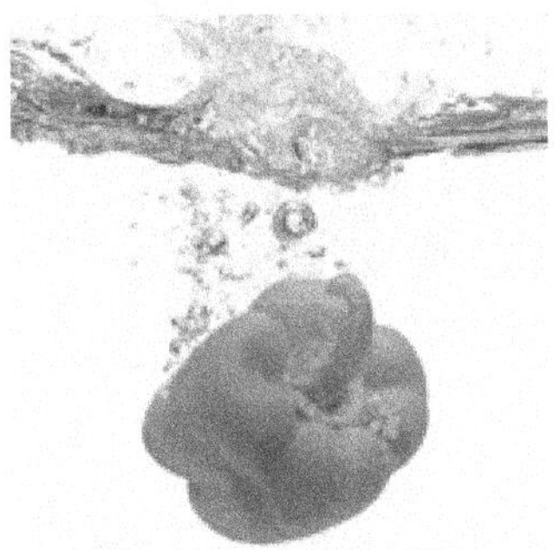

Grapefruit: this tangy, juicy fruit contains a water content of 90.5%. It burns fat, shrinks your waistline, and stabilizes blood sugar. Thus, plays a significant role towards the freshness of your skin.

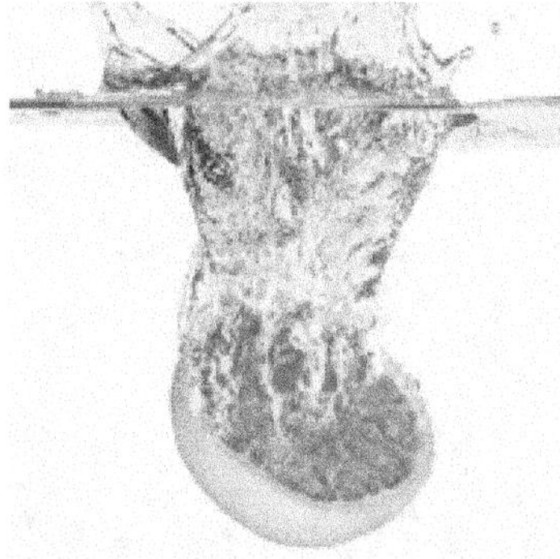

Strawberries: they have a water content of 91.0%. Blueberries and raspberries both hover more than 85% content of water in them.

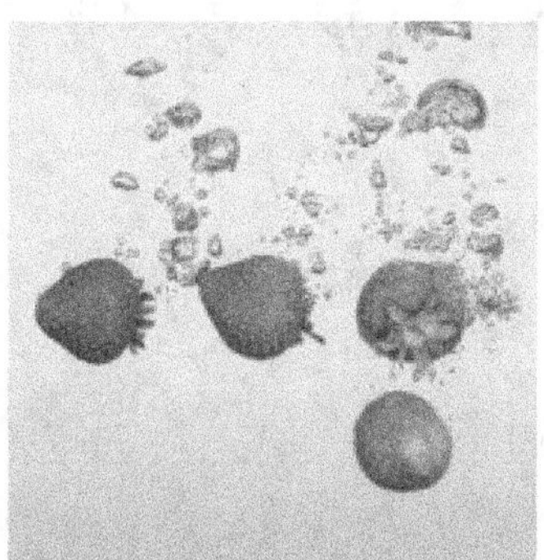

Iceberg Lettuce:

After cucumbers, it is the iceberg lattice that contains around 95.6% water is its structure. It contains a high amount of fibers as well. It is also rich in vitamin K and folate. You can use it in your sandwiches or as a bed for your evening salads.

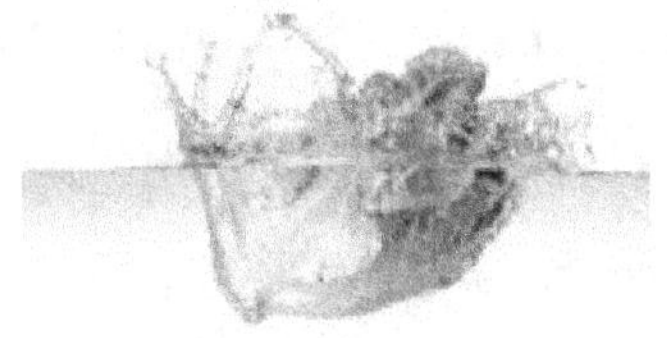

Chapter 2 – Tips to Get Rid of Cellulite with Water

Cellulite is not everyone's favorite topic. Some people might not like to talk about it due to its other names such as hail damage, orange peel, and cottage cheese thighs. People, especially women, avoid having a conversation on this topic because the vast majority of them have cottage cheese thighs!

At the same time, you must talk down to yourself. Loving your body is a big art. It does not matter if you have a few pockets and some dimples to spare on your thighs. You must always appreciate your body as it keeps you alive and does wonders for you.

The good news for you is that you can step ahead and reduce cellulite from your body. You may doubt it, but you can help your body to become leaner and firmer and reduce cellulite. But before that, you must know what cellulite is, why does it occur, and how can you reduce its appearance. Thus, you won't need to be bikini shame anymore!

Cellulite:

Fat loves to get deposited in your body. If it sits down right under your skin, naturally in the lower pelvic and the abdomen, then we name it cellulite like on buttocks and thighs.

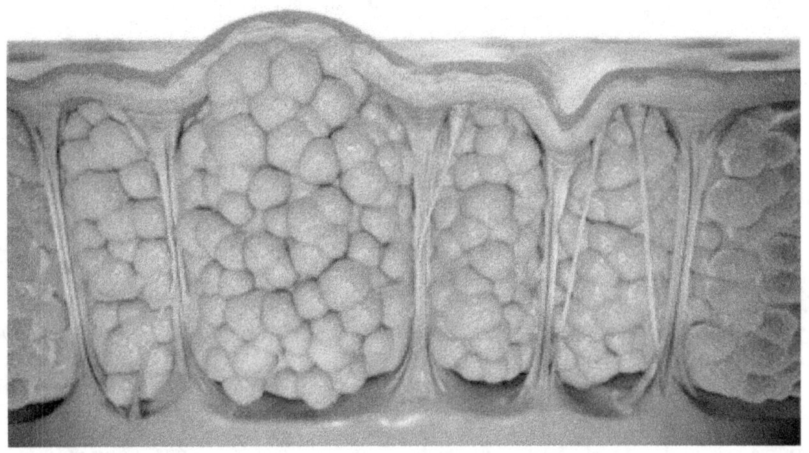

There are many contributors in the appearance of cellulite under your skin such as generic disposition, age, lifestyle choices, and poor diet. Each of the factors plays a significant role in accumulating the fats under your skin in your body in the form of cellulite. There is a common denominator for all these factors as well, and that is the toxicity that it causes by sitting on your thighs.

Cellulite is an accumulation of all the waste food such as preservatives, pesticides, chemicals, animal proteins, and quality food you have been eating over the past many years.

Next, come to the environmental pollutants and chemicals outside in the environment and inside your house. You are facing these pollutants for many years. You might have also consumed alcohol, have smoked and took drugs (pharmaceutical medicines included) for prolonged periods.

All of them sit down in your body and accumulate under your skin in the form of cellulite. These are the toxins that your body is unable to eliminate her. Also, you just keep on adding more waste products in your body without noticing the amount of the accumulated fats and their life-taking side effects.

Relation between Cellulite and Toxins

Toxins are accumulated in our bodies through the food that we eat. Our body is an ingenious mechanism. It stores these toxins within the fat accumulations around our muscles so that major body organs do not get exposed to the toxins much. That's why skinny persons with unhealthy lifestyles are more prone to infections and other diseases than the slightly overweight persons living with an unhealthy way of life.

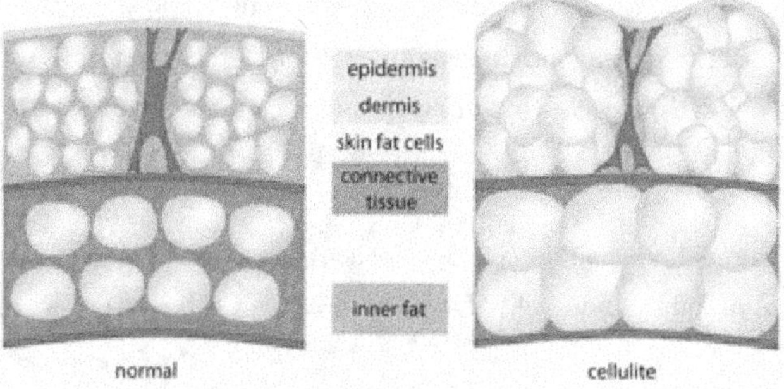

The slightly fat people contain that extra layer of fats along with the toxins in their bodies that prevent the other principal organs from coming into the direct contact with these toxins. Therefore, you must realize the fact the indentation and pockets located in your cellulite are also tempting places to store toxins of your body.

If you feel ashamed of these dimples on your thighs today, then you are not going to be jubilant with them after a few, say five, years when they would have gotten only worse. Ladies! It is the time to jump out of your bed and start working on reducing cellulite from your body.

Reducing Cellulite Using Water:

As we have already discussed the cellulite is nothing other than little fats. Therefore, you have to work hard to get rid of the buildup of toxins in your body. But you just can't stop at this step. You also need to prevent further accumulation as well.

There are many remedies for it. But what is the better option if you already have water available?! You must hydrate and flush your body more often to reduce and prevent the toxins accumulations in your body.

Hydrate and Flush:

Firstly, you need to drink lots of clean water. It keeps your body hydrated. Secondly, you must hydrate your body from fresh vegetables and fruits. It will allow flushing out of the toxins out of your physical body. Both of these steps work in correlation to each other.

Water is an essential element of our bodies. Most of the human body consists of it. Its deprivation in human body results in an ages, lumpy, and shriveled structure. Drinking lots of water will help you achieving a supple and smooth skin. And cellulite does not occur in such skins.

So, you can use water for dual benefits here, firstly for maintaining a beautiful skin, and secondly for preventing cellulite.

To have a healthy, cellulite free body, you must consume water early in the morning before taking breakfast. If you are that kind of person who does not like to drink lots of water, then you can add some lime juice in it. You can put lemon slices in it as well.

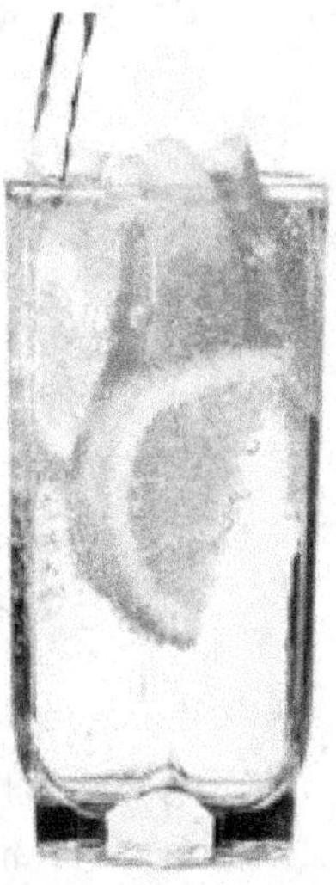

If you want to do more experiments with this morning water routine of yours, then you can go for herbal tea. But do not take coffee or black tea in the morning on empty stomach. These drinks dehydrate your body. If you are habitual of consuming such kind of drinks, then you must take lots of water during the day as well. It will maintain the level of hydration in your body.

Chapter 3 – Tips to Drink Water to Get Elasticity Back

Summer is the best time to talk about water. It is a season when the temperature climbs a mountain. Many people get in the emergency sections of the hospitals due to heat strokes. Muscles spasms start occurring more often as well. These stories just keep going.

The importance of water for our bodies increases in summers. Water is an essential element of our bodies. Most of the human body consists of it. An average human body is 80% water whereas the body muscles contain 75% of it.

This deprivation in human body results in an ages, lumpy, and shriveled structure. Therefore, the human body must always be kept hydrated. The muscles start losing their elasticity with the diminishing water content. With this worse development, the muscles get tight and might get spasms as well.

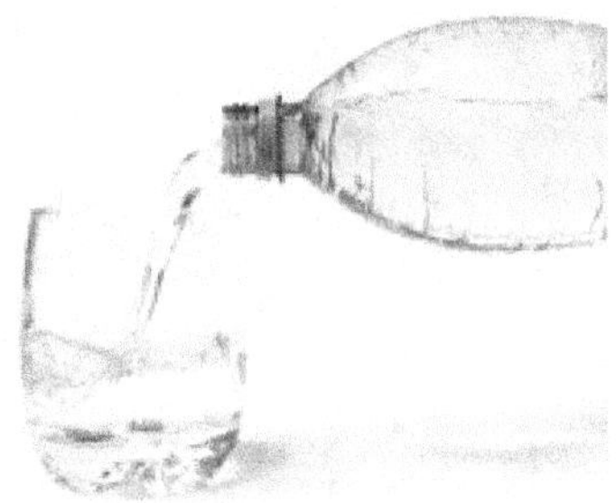

It is a crucial fact that most of the people on this planet are dehydrated, and they don't even realize it. They only drink when they are thirsty.

However, thirst is not the only sign of dehydration in your body. It may even not come on the second number as well. Following are some of the significant signs of dehydration in your body:

1. Anger

2. No tears when crying

3. Dizziness

4. Confusion

5. Sleepiness

6. Little or no urine

7. Dry mouth

8. Constipation

9. Headaches

10. Digestive discomfort

11. Fatigue

12. Etc.

Dehydration even can end up in more dangerous conditions as such;

1. Allergies

2. Asthma

3. Obesity

4. Ulcers

It is a common observation that elder people experience these symptoms more than the younger ones even at the same level of dehydration.

If after reading all these facts you have decided to drink more water then remember that you must only consume filtered or cleaned water.

Bottled water is the best option for you. You must at least drink ten to twelve glasses of water a day to maintain the hydration level in your body.

Let's read about what exactly the elasticity of muscles means:

Elasticity of the Muscles:

Elasticity is the ability to move your muscles in a comprehensive range of movements. Because of this elasticity, our bodies can move in various directions and carry numerous tasks. However, this elasticity can be restricted due to certain factors such as:

1. Restriction due to any equipment or clothing

2. Genders (females are more elastic than the males)

3. Age (Adults are less flexible than the pre-adolescents)

4. Any injury in the joint or muscle cramp

5. The time of the day (some people are more flexible in the morning, others in the evenings)

6. The temperature of the place (where you are at that moment)

7. Level of hydration in your body

Hydration: Why is it so Important:

Every organ, tissue, and cell of the human body require water to survive and to carry out the tasks correctly. For example, your body uses water to remove wastes, maintain its temperature, and lubricate the joints and hydrate the muscles. You are at higher risk to suffer from dehydration if:

1. You are trying to lose weight

2. You have been vomiting

3. You have diarrhea

4. You are suffering from fever

5. You are exercising

6. You are outside under direct sun

7. You are pregnant

8. You are breastfeeding

You have certain medical conditions such bladder infections or kidney stones

Therefore, you must keep your body hydrated all the time. You must drink lots of clean and filtered water.

Hydration and Elasticity of Your Body:

To maintain the elasticity of your body, you must consume at least ten to twelve glasses of water every day. It may sound like a daunting task to you. You cannot keep drinking water all the day. Therefore, you might think about eating your water!

Eat Your Water:

Yes, that's right! You can eat your water through various food items. Roughly 20% water of your daily routine comes from the solid food items. But it is still important to drink ample water, especially in the summer time.

Tips to Drink Water to Getting Elasticity Back:

1. Eat Cucumbers:

The water content of cucumber is 96.7%. It is the only solid food that contains this much water in it. You can serve it with hummus, eat in slices, or make part of a salad. You can even pump up its moisture content by blending it up with ice cubes, mint, and nonfat yogurt. It will make up soup for you. Soup is very hydrating, but the problem is that you might not like to have any hot thing in the summertime. But we have a solution for that as well! Put the cucumber soup in the refrigerator. Who doesn't like a chilled treat in summer?!

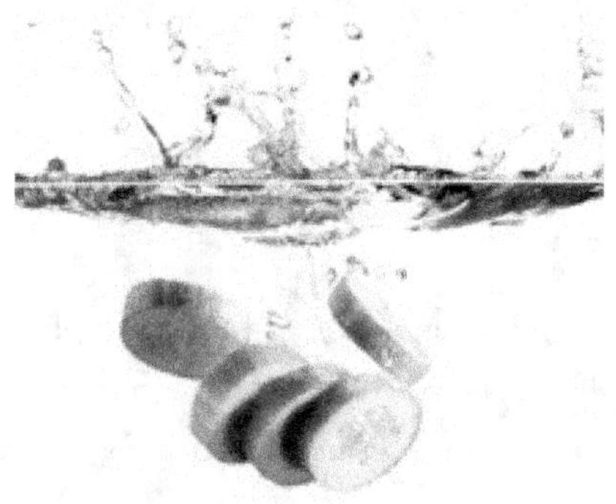

2.   Consume Iceberg Lettuce:

After cucumbers, it is the iceberg lattice that contains around 95.6% water is its structure. It contains a high amount of fibers as well. It is also rich in vitamin K and folate. You can use it in your sandwiches or as a bed for your evening salads.

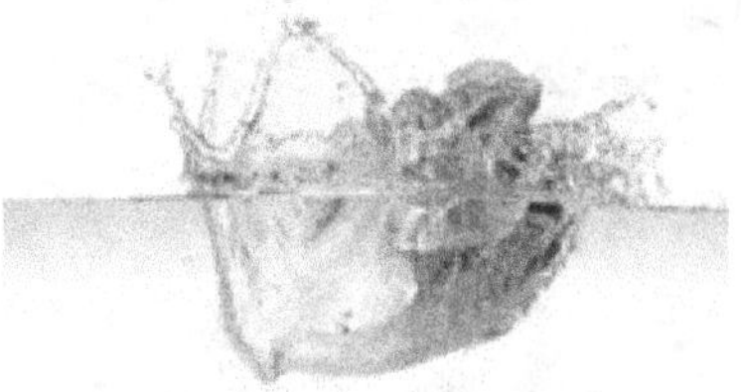

3.   Make Celery Your New Friend:

Celery has a water content of 95.4%. It only contains six calories per stalk. It is also rich in vitamins K, C, and A, and folate. It neutralizes the stomach and is considered as an excellent natural remedy for acid reflux and heartburn.

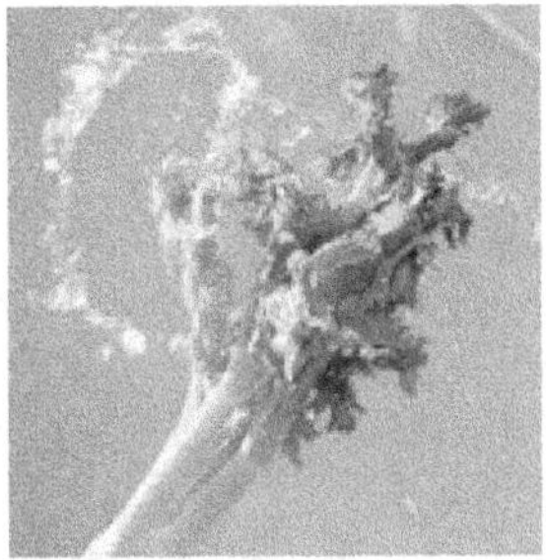

4. Take Radishes:

Radishes contain up to 95.3% water in their structures. It is a refreshing root vegetable. It contains a spicy-sweet flavor. It has a crunchy texture. It is a perfect addition in your nutritious summer coleslaw.

You can also make up a salad with it by adding parsley, chopped hazelnuts, sliced snow peas, and shredded carrots and cabbages, toss with salt, pepper, olive oil, lemon juice, and poppy seeds.

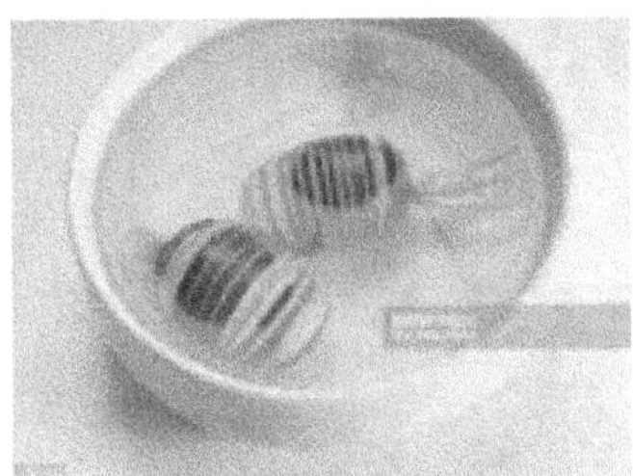

5. Munch Tomatoes:

Tomatoes contain 94.5% water. They are a mainstay of sandwiches, sauces, and salads. You can add grape varieties and sweet cherries to make up a nutritious salad for you with high water content.

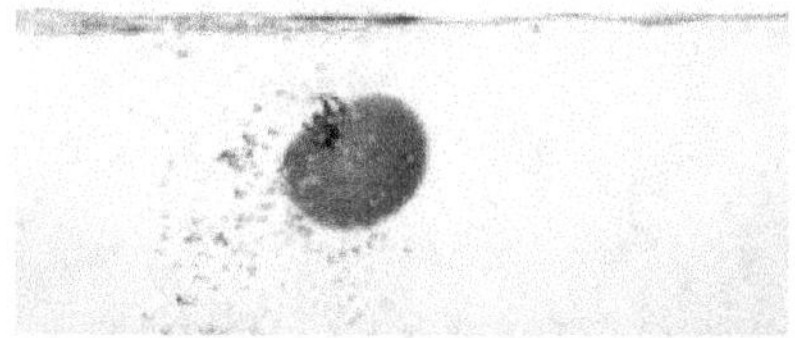

Chapter 4 – One Month Water Diet to Make Your Skin Fresh

Skincare is such a vast topic that most of the times that a lot of misinformation prevails in it. It's okay to get well-intentional bad advice on the subject from plenty of oil-wives. It happens because taking care of your skin is tricky. It also varies with every kind of skin. However, you can locate some basic tried and true rules in it as well. These rules usually falsify one or two of the pointers in your skin care notebook that you have already heard and believed.

Likewise, a regular day example on the topic includes the misconception about using hot water to wash your face as it is the better method to cleanse your skin thoroughly. However, this myth is not true. You do not need to wash your face with hot water to clean it. It can cause irritation and redness in people with sensitive skin.

And all the people out there with healthy skin may experience drying out their delicate facial skin with the use of hot water. It makes the skin more susceptible to all types of problems such as acne, flaky dermis, or redness. You must only use mildly warm to room-temperature water on your skin. It is enough to clean your pores without causing any irritation. Apply same rule on the whole of your skin, and do not restrict it to your face only.

You may enjoy burning your skin up in the hot shower with the imagination of deep cleaning it, but it makes it irritate and get red, especially as cool weather draws close.

What You Eat Matters for Your Skin:

Many people believe in applying various fruits and vegetables on their skins to nourish it which is a good practice and makes the skin healthier and more glowing. Along with it, what you eat also contributes towards the nourishment of your skin. That's why a healthy diet with lots of water, lot of fresh veggies and fruits, minimal alcohol, some skin-benefitting tea, and plenty of sweat drenching exercise made your skin glowing and cleaned more than any branded and expensive moisturizer and cleanser. It makes you feel great too.

One Month Water Diet to Make Your Skin Fresh:

Keeping your skin hydrated is pertinent especially in the winter seasons. It gets dry quickly with most of us not exercising much and all heaters pumping out dry air. It also makes us less mindful about drinking and consuming the required amount of water. Also, it is not possible to drink lots of liquids in winter which are essential to keep your skin happy and plump.

This kind of skin has a higher tolerance against the viruses and bacteria as well. Remember that dry mucous layer is vulnerable to the attacks due to the body's weak defense system. However, most of the time it is just too unappetizing and chilly to drink plain water all day long. Here, we are providing with a few food items and some skin benefitting teas that you can consume over a period of one month to deeply nourish your skin and make it glowing.

Morning Water Routine:

Taking one or two glasses of water on an empty stomach early in the morning is highly recommendable to get a flat stomach and refreshed skin.

Salad with High Content of Water:

To consume during the daytime, you can toss up a salad for you in which you include some of the following ingredients as they contain high water content:

Cucumbers: with a water content of 96.7%, cucumbers are highly hydrating. Dice or slice them and add to your salad.

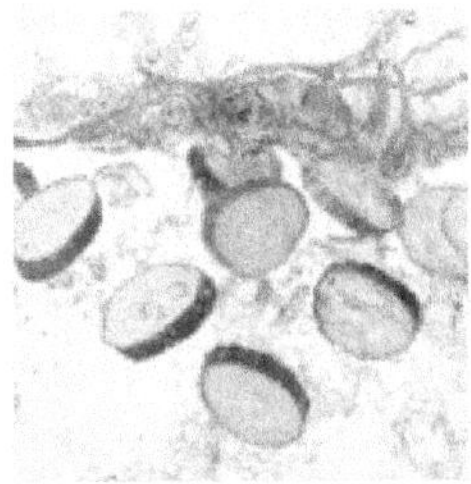

Radishes: they have a water content of 95.3%, they have a spicy-sweet taste and thus, makes an excellent addition to your salad plate.

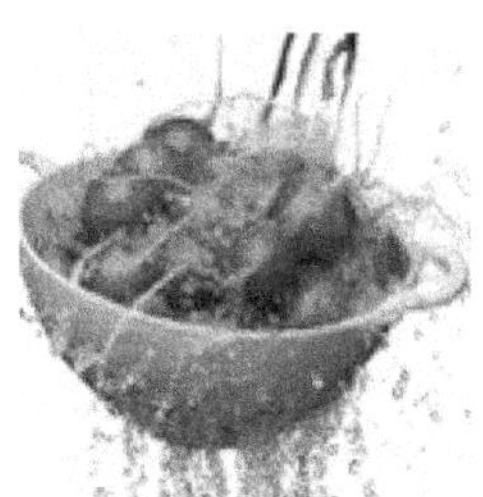

Tomatoes: they are all water with consistency level at 94.5%, take out their seeds before adding them to your salad.

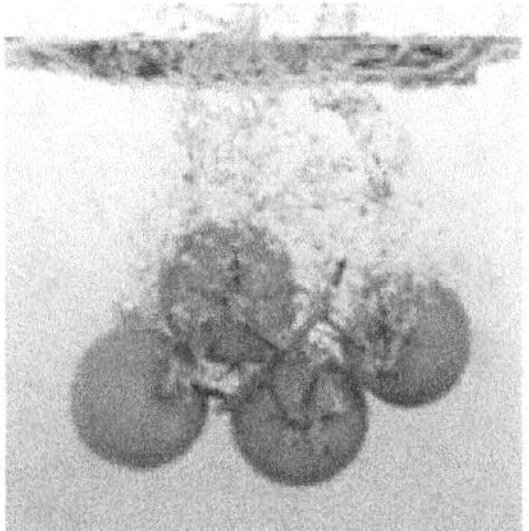

Green peppers: all bell peppers have high water texture, yet green bell peppers are on the top with 93.9% water content. They make a great addition to your salad with the sharp, hot taste.

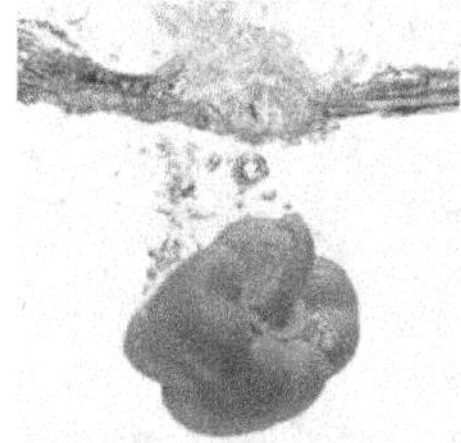

Spinach: it contains 91.4% water content. This leafy vegetable is an essential ingredient to keep your skin healthy and fresh when on a water diet.

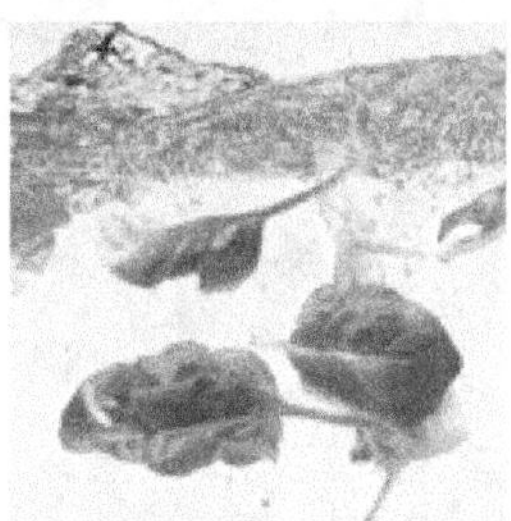

Baby Carrots: they are small but contain a water content of 90.4%. Slice and add them to your salad.

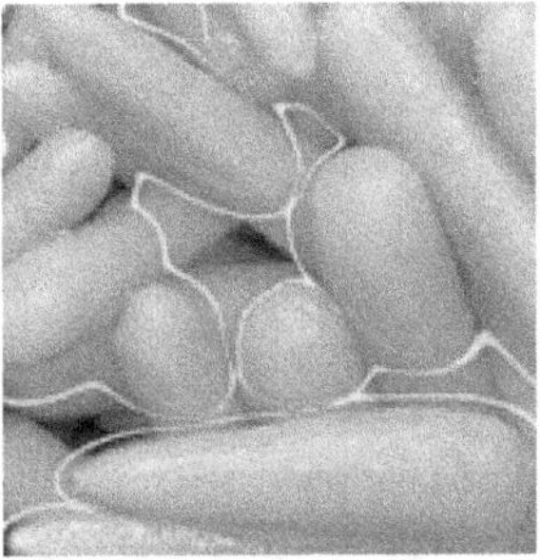

Consuming Fresh Fruits and Veggies:

If you are on a one-month water diet to make your skin clean, then the goal cannot be achieved without consuming lots of raw fruits and vegetables. You must go for the seasonal veggies and fruits. However, here is a list of certain greens for you:

Cantaloupe: its water content is 90.2%. It is succulent watermelon. It is an excellent source of water with a few calories. It is also enriched with vitamins A and C that play a significant role in refreshing your skin.

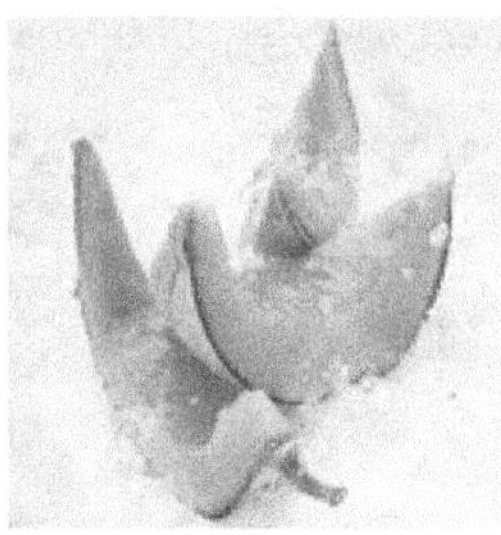

Grapefruit: this tangy, juicy fruit contains a water content of 90.5%. It burns fat, shrinks your waistline, and stabilizes blood sugar. Thus, plays a significant role towards the freshness of your skin.

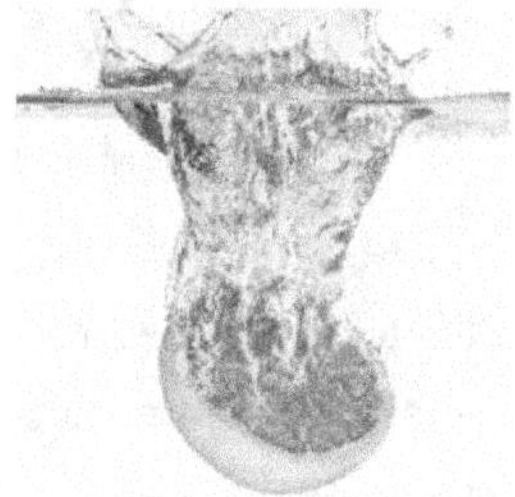

Broccoli: with a water content of 90.7% broccoli is enriched with vitamin C and A, potassium and fiber.

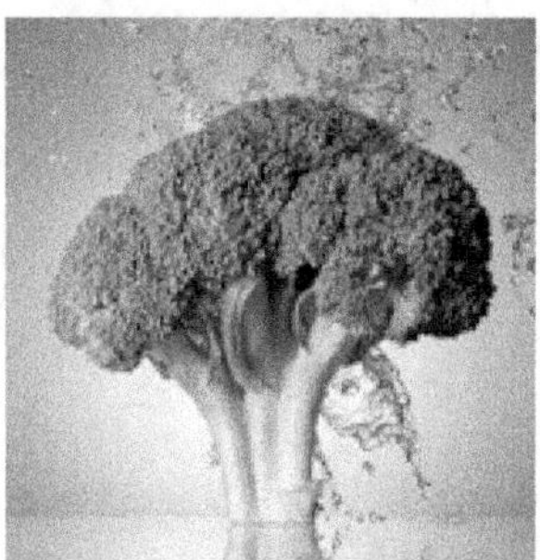

Strawberries: they have a water content of 91.0%. Blueberries and raspberries both hover more than 85% content of water in them.

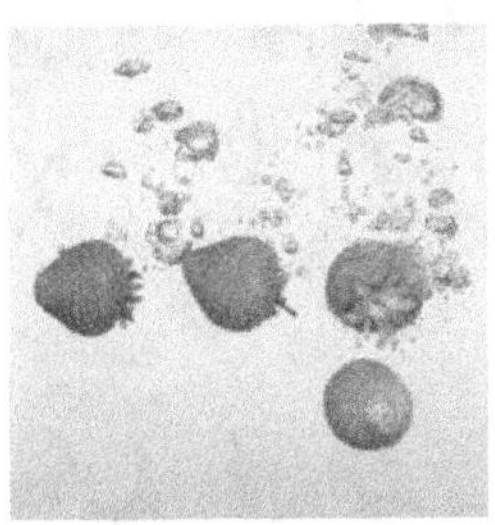

Watermelon: with a water content of 91.5%, watermelon is all water. It highly hydrates your skin.

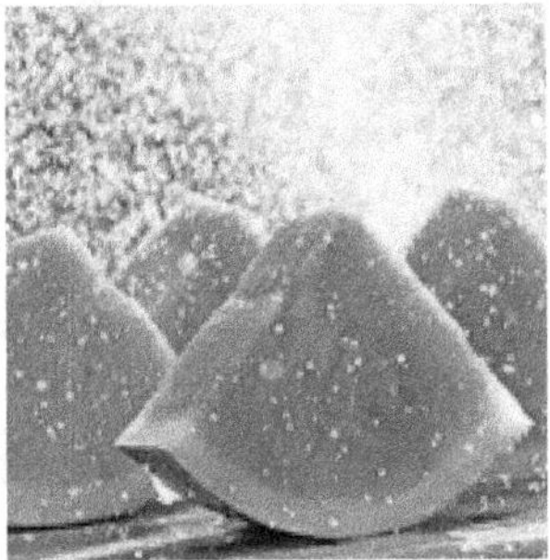

Cauliflower: it contains 92.1% water in it. It is packed with phytonutrients and vitamins.

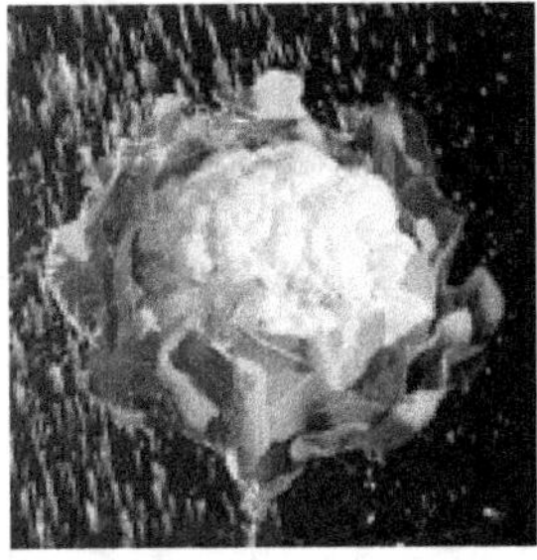

Celery: it contains 95.4% water in it. It has only six calories per stalk. It highly hydrates your body and skin.

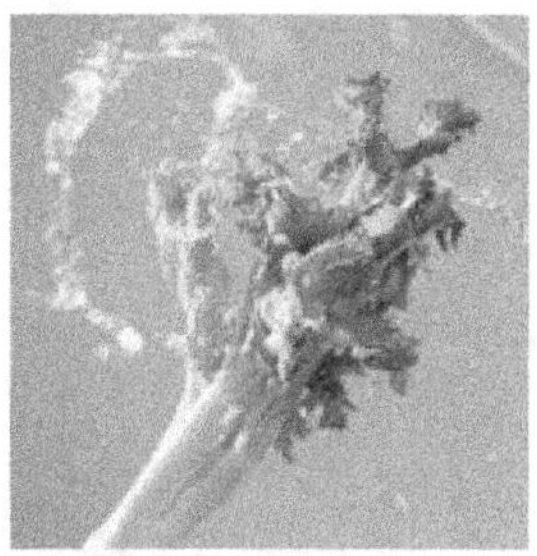

Iceberg Lettuce: with 95.6% water content, it is enriched with vitamin k and folate.

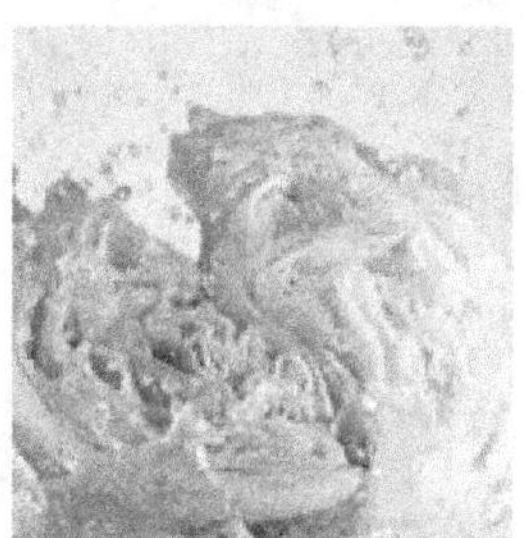

Chapter 5 – Proven Methods to Reduce Weight without Dieting and with Water

Most of the people want to reduce their weight without dieting because it is hard to stick to an exercise plan and a conventional diet program. For all of you, there are several proven techniques and methods to reduce weight this way. These programs help you consuming mindlessly fewer calories. These methods and ways not only reduce your current weight but also prevent your body from putting on the weight again in the future.

In this chapter, we are discussing proven methods to shed your body weight without adopting any particular diet plan and consuming more water than regular. Let's read together!

Method # 01: Drink Water Regularly:

You must drink water daily. It is good for both your skin and body. It fills your stomach and makes you eat less especially if you are regular in taking it before your meal every day. Thus, you start losing weight without holding up to any particular diet plan.

One scientific study on the adults showed that consuming almost half a liter of water half an hour before the meal reduced the hunger in the subjects and thus, they consumed fewer amounts of calories. These subjects, to be precise, lost 44% more water with this essential water drinking technique over a period of twelve weeks than the uncontrolled subjects.

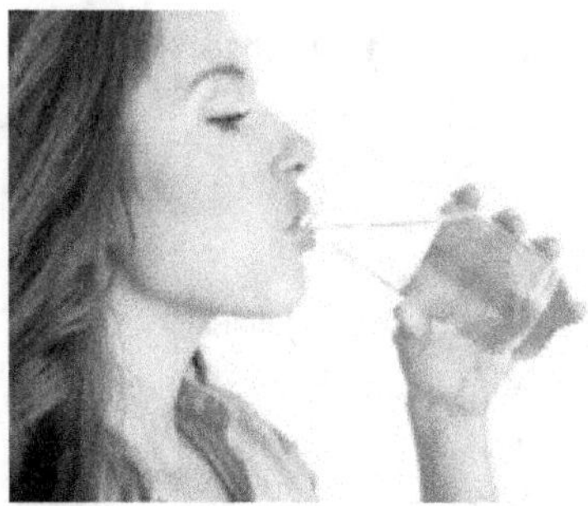

Even, if you find it difficult to consume half glass of water half hour before your meal every time, you can replace the calorie-loaded drinks such as juice or soda with a plain glass of water. It will start showing miraculous effects in a short while.

Bottom line: Drink water before the meal to reduce weight without dieting. Replacing calorie-loaded drinks with plain water is beneficial.

Method # 02: Chew Thoroughly and Slow Down:

It is pertinent to make your brain realize that you have had enough to eat. It takes time in processing this information. If you chew your food slow, it will provide your brain to process the information. It also makes you eat slowly.

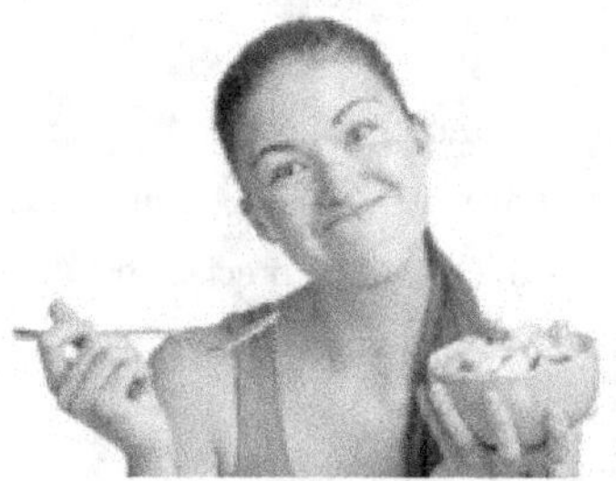

Thus, you intake less food, fullness is increased, and smaller portions are attained. All of these steps help you reducing weight without adopting any particular diet plan.

Bottom line: Eating slow makes you feel filled sooner than otherwise.

Method # 03: Use Small Plates for Unhealthy Food:

A few decades ago, the serving plate was much smaller than it is today. It is unfortunate. Apparently, we eat more on a large plate. Small plate makes the food appear huge, and you unconsciously get satisfied with the amount of food and thus, consume less.

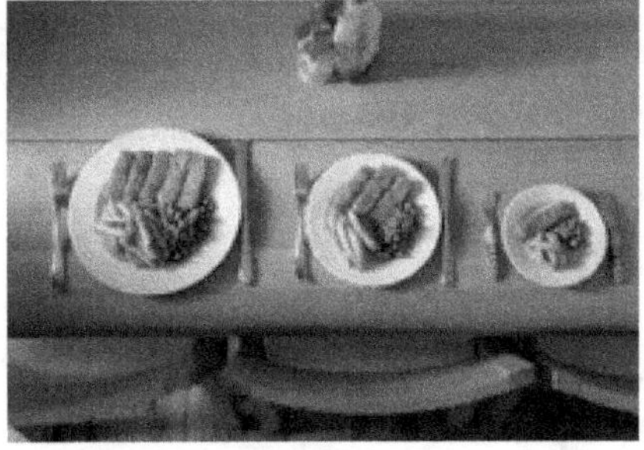

 On the contrary, a large plate makes the food seem less and insufficient for your stomach to become happy with.

Bottom line: Small plates trick your brain to think the food is enough. Large plates increase the amount intake of food.

Method # 04: Serve Yourself Smaller Portions:

Over the last few decades, along with the plates, the size of servings has increased as well. This tradition makes us consume more than the required amount of food, particularly in the restaurants. It is not a good habit. Thus, it is pertinent to serve yourself smaller portions of food throughout the day.

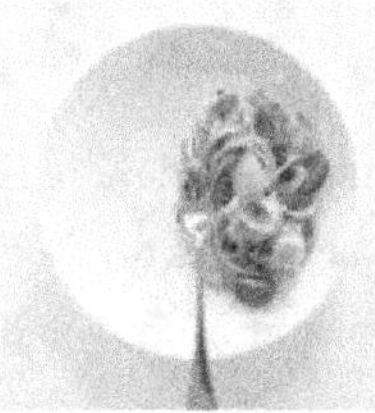

One scientific study has proven that the larger sizes of plates make you consume about 30% more than the required amount of calories per day. It is for the same reason that obesity is much prevalent in the present generation of the humans.

If you serve yourself small portions of food, you will not eat less, but your brain will also not realize the trick and the stomach will get filled quickly. It is a great strategy to consume less and reduce weight without any dieting.

Bottom line: Trick your mind by serving yourself small portions of food throughout the day.

Method # 05: Eat Without Electronic Devices:

The modern era is plentiful of electronic devices. Everyone has some gadget in his hand while eating. This habit takes away your attention from your food which makes you consume more than the required amount of food.

Paying attention to your food may help you in consuming lesser calories. Do not eat your meal while you are playing computer games or watching TV. You will lose the track of what you are entering in your body this way.

Twenty-four scientific studies were carried, and one review article of them concluded that people who consumed their food while using any electronic gadget took in 10% more than their regular food in that one particular sitting.

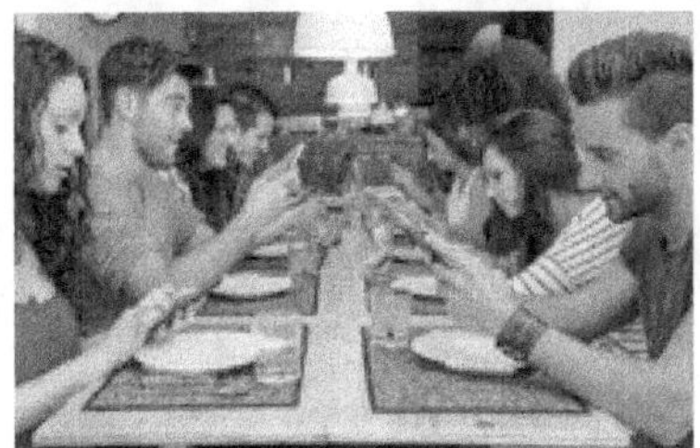

It does not stop here. Another study has shown that taking meals while surfing on the electronic appliances make you take more food later in the day. The food that you consume without paying attention to it does not get registered by your brain. Thus, your stomach automatically runs the signal of being empty just after a short while of taking the meal. You start feeling hungry again and thus, take another meal.

In this way, you not consume more while not paying attention to your food at the first place and then consume more food later because your brain was unable to register the intake. It increases your body weight.

Bottom line: Consuming food while distracted results in consuming more calories. Paying attention while eating helps you in reducing weight by consuming less in the first place.

Conclusion

Every organ, tissue, and cell of the human body requires water to survive and to carry out the tasks correctly. Drinking lots of organic, clean water is an inevitable part of maintaining both of your health and skin.

Dehydrated skin also does not have the ability to repair itself. Also, it is unable to generate new cells. It results in the appearance of the signs of aging in human bodies. Thus, hydrating your body can reduce these effects. You must hydrate your skin from inside and outside.

Experts recommend an average human being to consume more or less eight glasses of pure organic and clean water every day. However, your body may demand more water if you sweat a lot, or you are exercising.

You must take a balanced diet to maintain the glow and freshness of your skin. It includes the proper amount of fresh fruits and vegetables, a certain amount of proteins and lots of water.

FREE Bonus Reminder

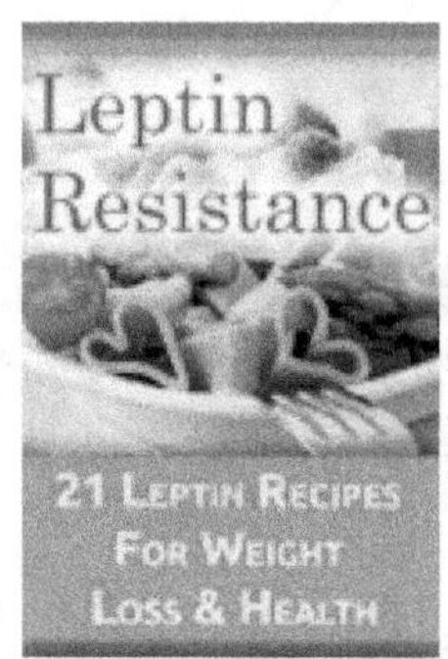

If you have not grabbed it yet, please go ahead and download your special bonus report *"Leptin Resistance. 21 Leptin Recipes For Weight Loss & Healthy Living"*.

Simply Click the Button Below

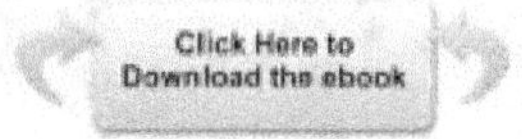

OR **Go to This Page**

http://easyweightlossway.com/free/

BONUS #2: More Free & Discounted Books

Do you want to receive more Free & Discounted Books?

We have a mailing list where we send out our new Books when they go free or with a discount on Kindle. Click on the link below to sign up for Free & Discount Book Promotions.

=> Sign Up for Free & Discount Book Promotions <=

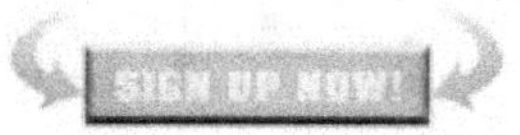

OR Go to this URL

http://zbit.ly/1WBb1Ek

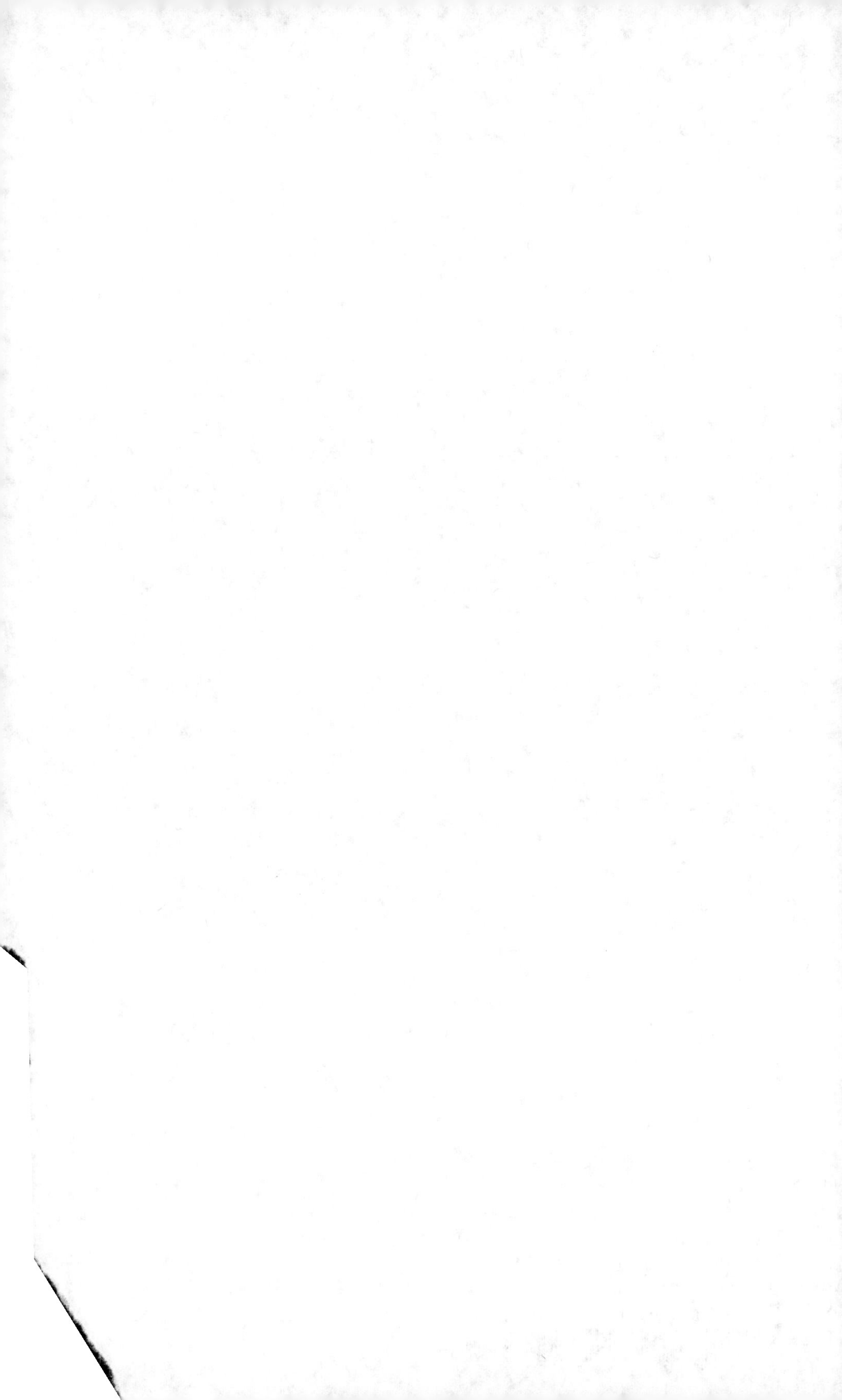